# Recharge: The Silent Power of Sleep

# Dedication

To my parents,
For your unwavering love, guidance,
and belief in me.


And to my sister,
For always standing by my side with
encouragement and support.


Thank you for being my greatest
pillars of strength.


This journey wouldn't have
been possible without you.

*Sometimes, a little space is all we need—
this page is intentionally left blank.*

# Recharge: The Silent Power of Sleep

ROHAN SAHOO

# Recharge: The Silent Power of Sleep

## Book Details

Title: - **Recharge: The Silent Power of Sleep**

Author: **Rohan Sahoo**

Genre: **Psychology / Health & Wellness**

Publisher: Rohan Sahoo

Pages: 80

Cover Image by: **Fidan Nazim Qizi**

Format: Available in eBook formats

# Book Description

In **The Sleep Revolution: Unlocking the Power of Rest**, author Rohan Sahoo takes readers on an enlightening journey into one of the most overlooked aspects of health and well-being: sleep. In a society that glorifies productivity and long work hours, sleep is often sacrificed, seen as a luxury rather than a necessity. Rohan challenges this notion, shedding light on the profound impact that quality sleep has on every aspect of our lives, from our physical and mental health to our productivity and emotional resilience.

Drawing on the latest research in psychology, neuroscience, and sleep science, *The Sleep Revolution* explores the powerful relationship between sleep and overall health. Rohan explains how disrupted sleep can lead to issues like weakened immune response, mental fatigue, memory loss, and mood disorders, impacting our ability to function effectively each day. By outlining the biological mechanisms of sleep, the book provides readers with a scientific foundation for understanding why sleep is essential and how lack of it can hinder personal growth, success, and well-being.

What sets *The Sleep Revolution* apart is its actionable guidance based on the principles of the **8×3 Law—a time management framework** designed to help individuals structure their day around productive work intervals while ensuring adequate time for rest. Rohan introduces readers to the 8×3 Law as *a tool for achieving balance between work, rest, and personal activities, encouraging readers to allocate specific blocks of time for restorative sleep*. The *8×3 Law will* reinforce the importance of regular rest intervals and emphasizes the benefits of high-quality sleep in making productive use of our waking hours.

Each chapter of this book is dedicated to a specific aspect of sleep, from the science of circadian rhythms and the impact of screen time to strategies for combating insomnia and establishing bedtime routines. Readers will learn about the common obstacles that interfere with sleep, such as stress, inconsistent schedules, and environmental factors, and will discover practical techniques to counter these challenges. He offers simple, sustainable solutions for creating a sleep-friendly environment, including tips on managing light exposure, reducing noise, and optimizing bedroom comfort. By implementing these practices, readers can cultivate healthier sleep habits and make lasting improvements to their overall lifestyle.

Beyond the science, *The Sleep Revolution* also delves into the psychological and emotional dimensions of sleep. Rohan discusses how anxiety, depression, and even social pressures can disrupt our sleep patterns and explores the ways that mindful practices—like relaxation exercises, gratitude journaling, and deep breathing techniques—can alleviate these disruptions. By addressing these psychological factors, the book empowers readers to approach sleep not only as a physical need but as a holistic experience that requires attention to both the mind and body.

Rohan's approach is practical, accessible, and filled with empathy for readers navigating the demands of modern life. Throughout the book, he emphasizes that improving sleep is not about aiming for perfection but about making small, realistic changes that lead to big improvements over time. With easy-to-follow advice, real-life examples, and reflective exercises, *The Sleep Revolution* serves as a personalized guide for anyone seeking to transform their relationship with sleep.

By prioritizing sleep as a crucial aspect of personal development, *The Sleep Revolution* empowers readers to experience the life-altering benefits of proper rest. As Rohan eloquently explains, a well-rested mind is more creative, a well-rested body is more resilient, and a well-rested soul is more fulfilled. Whether you're a student, a professional, a parent, or simply someone struggling with poor sleep, this book will inspire you to reclaim your nights and unlock your full potential by embracing the power of rest.

This book is an invitation to redefine how we view sleep and to recognize it as an essential component of a thriving, successful life. By the end of *The Sleep Revolution*, readers will have the tools, insights, and motivation to make sleep a priority, allowing them to approach each day with renewed energy, focus, and purpose.

# TO,
## MY BEST FRIEND,

## SLEEP.

# Table of Contents

## **Target Audience**

This book is intended for anyone looking to improve their sleep quality and overall health, including:

- Individuals struggling with sleep issues
- Students and professionals seeking to enhance their productivity
- Parents aiming to establish healthy sleep routines for their children
- Anyone interested in psychology, health, and wellness

## **Additional Resources**

Readers will find valuable resources, including:

- Sleep habit checklists
- Relaxation and mindfulness exercises
- Links to further reading and research studies
- A dedicated online community for sharing experiences and tips on improving sleep habits

# Preface

In today's fast-paced world, sleep is often treated as an afterthought—a luxury we indulge in only when absolutely necessary. Many of us sacrifice precious hours of rest for work, social obligations, or screen time, not realizing the cost this has on our health, productivity, and happiness. *Recharge: The Silent Power of Sleep* was born from a simple yet profound realization: sleep is not just a state of rest but a cornerstone of a fulfilling life.

As I navigated my own journey of personal development, I discovered that mastering time management and achieving balance were impossible without prioritizing quality sleep. This book aims to provide a comprehensive look into the science of sleep, the psychological factors that influence our sleep patterns, and practical strategies to build a sustainable, healthy sleep routine.

With insights (soon to be published) grounded in research and the principles of the 8×3 Law—a time management method that emphasizes the importance of completing essential tasks in structured intervals—I hope to guide readers toward making sleep a priority.

Throughout this book, I share techniques that anyone can incorporate into their daily lives, regardless of lifestyle or schedule. I've combined advice from psychologists, sleep researchers, and wellness experts with practical exercises to help you overcome sleep-related obstacles. By taking small, manageable steps, you can improve your quality of life and approach each day with renewed energy and focus.

This book is for anyone who wants to regain control of their sleep, enhance their well-being, and experience the transformative power of rest. My hope is that as you read these pages, you'll begin to view sleep not as a mere necessity, but as a powerful tool for achieving a healthier, more balanced life.

— *Rohan Sahoo*

# Recharge:
# The Silent Power of Sleep

ROHAN SAHOO

# Chapter 1: Introduction to Sleep Psychology

Sleep is a universal experience yet often undervalued in its importance to our overall health and well-being. In a fast-paced world that celebrates productivity and constant connectivity, sleep can easily become a casualty of our busy lives. Yet, the significance of sleep transcends mere rest; it is a complex process intricately linked to our physical, mental, and emotional health.

## Importance of Sleep

Research consistently shows that sleep is crucial for maintaining optimal health. According to the National Sleep Foundation, adults typically require 7 to 9 hours of sleep per night. Insufficient sleep can lead to a myriad of health issues, including obesity, diabetes, cardiovascular disease, and even early mortality. The World Health Organization identifies sleep as a fundamental human need, comparable to nutrition and exercise.

The consequences of inadequate sleep extend beyond physical health. Psychologically, sleep deprivation can impair cognitive functions such as attention, decision-making, and problem-solving. Chronic sleep deprivation has been linked to increased risk for mood disorders, including anxiety and depression. The relationship between sleep and mental health is cyclical; poor sleep can exacerbate psychological distress, while psychological stress can lead to disrupted sleep. This interdependence underscores the importance of prioritizing sleep in our daily routines.

Furthermore, sleep plays a vital role in cognitive functions such as memory consolidation, learning, problem-solving, and creativity. During sleep, especially during REM (Rapid Eye Movement) sleep, our brains process and organize the information we have gathered throughout the day. This is a period when the brain actively consolidates memories and integrates new knowledge with existing information. Dr. Matthew Walker, a neuroscientist and author of "Why We Sleep," states, "Sleep is the single most effective thing we can do to reset our brain and body health each day." This highlights not only the restorative nature of sleep but also its critical role in mental acuity and emotional stability.

In addition, sleep is essential for physical health. It influences metabolic functions, immune response, and the body's ability to repair itself. For example, during deep sleep, the body releases growth hormones that aid in tissue growth and muscle repair. Insufficient sleep has been shown to disrupt the balance of hormones that regulate appetite, leading to weight gain and increased cravings for unhealthy foods. This intricate connection between sleep and metabolism illustrates how vital restful nights are to maintaining a healthy weight and preventing lifestyle-related diseases.

## Overview of Sleep Stages

Sleep is not a uniform state; it consists of distinct stages that cycle throughout the night. These stages are divided into non-REM (NREM) and REM sleep. NREM sleep comprises three stages, each deeper than the last.

- Stage 1 (N1): This is the lightest stage of sleep, lasting only a few minutes. During this phase, the transition from wakefulness to sleep occurs, and the body begins to relax. People in this stage can be easily awakened and may experience drifting thoughts or sensations.

- Stage 2 (N2): This stage lasts for about 20 minutes and marks the onset of true sleep. Heart rate slows, body temperature decreases, and brain waves begin to show bursts of activity known as sleep spindles. This stage is crucial for learning and memory consolidation.

- Stage 3 (N3): Also known as deep sleep or slow-wave sleep, this stage is essential for physical recovery and health. The body is less responsive to external stimuli, making it difficult to wake someone in this stage. Growth hormones are released, and tissue repair occurs, emphasizing the restorative aspect of this sleep phase.

REM sleep, often associated with vivid dreaming, is where the brain is highly active. This stage is essential for emotional regulation and cognitive functions. During REM sleep, the brain processes emotions and experiences, aiding in problem-solving and creativity. The entire sleep cycle lasts about 90 minutes, and a healthy adult typically experiences 4 to 6 cycles per night, alternating between NREM and REM stages.

The intricate dance between sleep stages illustrates how essential sleep is for holistic health. Each stage has unique benefits and contributes to our overall psychological and physiological well-being. It is during these cycles that the brain and body restore, rejuvenate, and prepare for the challenges of the following day.

### The Societal Implications of Sleep Deprivation

In contemporary society, the cultural perception of sleep has evolved, often viewing it as a luxury rather than a necessity. Many individuals prioritize work, social engagements, and entertainment over sufficient rest, leading to a widespread culture of sleep deprivation. The American Psychological Association reports that nearly one-third of adults' report that they regularly do not get enough sleep, raising concerns about the long-term consequences of sleep deficiency.

Workplaces are increasingly recognizing the importance of sleep, understanding that productivity and creativity suffer when employees are fatigued. Initiatives such as flexible work hours, nap rooms, and sleep education programs are being implemented to promote healthier sleep habits among employees. As psychologist Dr. Dan P. Cohen notes, "The best way to predict your future is to create it," emphasizing the need for proactive measures to foster a culture that values sleep as an essential component of success.

## Conclusion 1

In conclusion, understanding sleep from a psychological perspective reveals its intricate connections to our overall health and functioning. Sleep is not merely a passive state but an active process that supports our physical, mental, and emotional well-being. As we continue to explore the complexities of sleep, it becomes increasingly clear that prioritizing rest is essential for achieving a balanced and fulfilling life. This chapter sets the foundation for further exploration into the science of sleep, the disorders that disrupt it, and the practical strategies we can employ to improve our sleep hygiene and, consequently, our overall quality of life.

# SLEEP STAGES

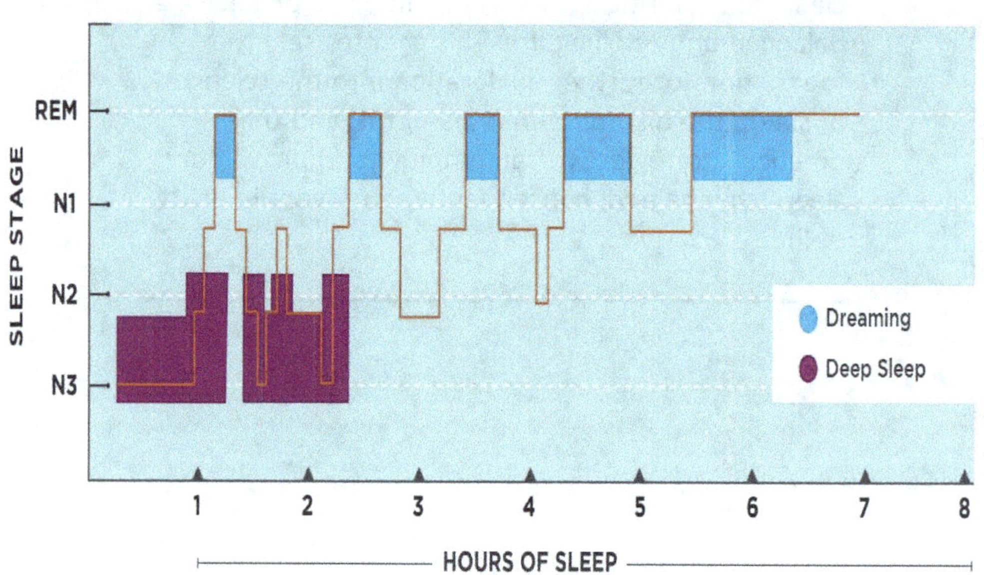

# Chapter 2: The Science of Sleep

Understanding the science of sleep is crucial for grasping its profound effects on our physical and psychological health. Sleep is a complex physiological process that involves various biological systems, including neurochemistry, circadian rhythms, and sleep architecture. This chapter delves into these components, exploring how they interact to regulate sleep and impact our overall well-being.

## Neurotransmitters and Hormones

At the heart of sleep regulation are neurotransmitters—chemical messengers that transmit signals in the brain. Several key neurotransmitters play vital roles in sleep regulation:

- GABA (Gamma-Aminobutyric Acid): This neurotransmitter promotes sleep by inhibiting neural activity. It reduces the overall excitability of neurons, helping to facilitate the transition from wakefulness to sleep. Many sleep medications work by enhancing GABA's effects, demonstrating its central role in sleep onset.

- Serotonin: Often referred to as the "feel-good" neurotransmitter, serotonin is also involved in regulating sleep-wake cycles. It is a precursor to melatonin, a hormone that signals the body when it's time to sleep. Proper serotonin levels are essential for maintaining healthy sleep patterns.

- Melatonin: Known as the sleep hormone, melatonin is produced by the pineal gland in response to darkness. It helps regulate circadian rhythms, signaling to the body that it is time to prepare for sleep. Melatonin levels typically rise in the evening and fall in the morning, creating a natural sleep-wake cycle. Supplementing melatonin can be beneficial for individuals with disrupted sleep patterns, such as shift workers or those experiencing jet lag.

- Cortisol: This hormone, often associated with stress, plays a role in regulating sleep as well. Cortisol levels typically rise in the morning, promoting alertness, and decrease throughout the day. Chronic stress can lead to elevated cortisol levels, disrupting the natural sleep cycle and contributing to insomnia.

Understanding how these neurotransmitters and hormones interact provides insight into the mechanisms behind sleep regulation and highlights the complexity of sleep physiology. Disruptions in any of these systems can lead to sleep disturbances and a host of related health issues.

### Circadian Rhythms

Circadian rhythms are natural, internal processes that follow a roughly 24-hour cycle, influencing various biological functions, including the sleep-wake cycle. The primary regulator of circadian rhythms is the suprachiasmatic nucleus (SCN), a group of nerve cells in the hypothalamus that respond to light and darkness cues. The SCN synchronizes the body's biological clock with the external environment, primarily influenced by light exposure.

Light exposure, particularly blue light from screens, can significantly impact circadian rhythms. Modern lifestyles often involve prolonged screen time, particularly in the evening, which can inhibit melatonin production and disrupt sleep patterns. Dr. PhD Mariana G. Figueiro, a researcher at the Lighting Research Center, states, "Light is the primary cue for our circadian rhythm, and understanding this relationship can help us mitigate sleep issues."

Maintaining a consistent sleep schedule, minimizing light exposure in the evening, and seeking natural light exposure during the day can help regulate circadian rhythms and improve sleep quality. Understanding these rhythms empowers individuals to make informed choices that support healthy sleep habits.

### Sleep Architecture

Sleep architecture refers to the structure and pattern of sleep cycles throughout the night. A typical sleep cycle consists of a progression through NREM and REM sleep stages, occurring several times throughout the night.

- NREM Sleep: As discussed in Chapter 1, NREM sleep consists of three stages, each contributing to physical restoration and memory consolidation. Deep sleep (Stage 3) is particularly important for bodily repair and immune function.

- REM Sleep: REM sleep is characterized by rapid eye movements, increased brain activity, and vivid dreaming. This stage is crucial for emotional regulation, creativity, and memory processing. The brain is busy during REM sleep, and it is during this time that emotional experiences are processed and integrated into long-term memory.

Healthy sleep architecture includes adequate amounts of both NREM and REM sleep. Disruptions to this architecture, such as sleep fragmentation or insufficient REM sleep, can lead to cognitive deficits, emotional instability, and overall diminished health.

### Sleep Disorders

Understanding the science of sleep also involves recognizing the various disorders that can disrupt healthy sleep patterns. Common sleep disorders include:

- Insomnia: Characterized by difficulty falling or staying asleep, insomnia can be caused by stress, anxiety, medical conditions, or poor sleep hygiene. Cognitive Behavioral Therapy for Insomnia (CBT-I) is an effective treatment that focuses on changing thoughts and behaviors surrounding sleep.

- Sleep Apnea: A serious disorder where breathing repeatedly stops and starts during sleep, sleep apnea can lead to fragmented sleep and daytime fatigue. It is often treated with lifestyle changes, continuous positive airway pressure (CPAP) therapy, or surgery.

- Restless Legs Syndrome (RLS): This neurological condition causes uncomfortable sensations in the legs and an irresistible urge to move them, particularly at night. Treatments may include lifestyle changes, medication, and supplements.

- Narcolepsy: A chronic sleep disorder characterized by excessive daytime sleepiness and sudden sleep attacks; narcolepsy can significantly impact daily functioning. Treatments often include medications and lifestyle adjustments.

Recognizing these disorders is crucial for seeking appropriate treatment and improving overall sleep quality. Understanding the science behind these conditions empowers individuals to advocate for their sleep health and explore potential interventions.

**Conclusion 2**

In conclusion, the science of sleep encompasses a multitude of biological processes that interact to regulate our sleep patterns. Understanding the role of neurotransmitters, circadian rhythms, sleep architecture, and sleep disorders provides valuable insights into how we can optimize our sleep and, consequently, our overall health. As we delve deeper into the intricacies of sleep psychology, we will explore practical strategies for enhancing sleep quality, addressing common sleep disturbances, and fostering a culture that prioritizes the essential nature of restorative sleep.

# Chapter 3: Common Sleep Disorders

Sleep disorders affect millions of individuals worldwide, often leading to serious health implications and diminished quality of life. Understanding these disorders, their symptoms, causes, and treatments is essential for promoting healthy sleep habits. In this chapter, we will explore several prevalent sleep disorders, shedding light on their characteristics and providing insights into effective management strategies.

## 1. Insomnia

Definition and Symptoms
Insomnia is characterized by difficulty falling asleep, staying asleep, or waking up too early without the ability to return to sleep. Individuals suffering from insomnia may experience daytime fatigue, irritability, and difficulty concentrating. Chronic insomnia is often defined as having difficulty sleeping at least three times per week for three months or longer.

Causes
The causes of insomnia are varied and can include psychological factors (like anxiety and depression), medical conditions (such as chronic pain or respiratory issues), lifestyle choices (like caffeine and alcohol consumption), and poor sleep hygiene. Stressful life events or changes, such as job loss, divorce, or the death of a loved one, can also trigger insomnia.

Treatment
Effective treatment for insomnia often includes a

combination of cognitive behavioral therapy (CBT) and lifestyle changes. CBT-I is a structured program that helps individuals identify and replace thoughts and behaviors that cause or worsen sleep problems. Sleep hygiene practices, such as maintaining a consistent sleep schedule, creating a relaxing bedtime routine, and optimizing the sleep environment, are crucial for improving sleep quality.

## 2. Sleep Apnea

Definition and Symptoms
Sleep apnea is a serious sleep disorder that occurs when breathing repeatedly stops and starts during sleep. The most common form is obstructive sleep apnea (OSA), where the throat muscles relax excessively during sleep, blocking the airway. Symptoms include loud snoring, choking or gasping during sleep, excessive daytime sleepiness, and difficulty concentrating.

Causes
Risk factors for sleep apnea include obesity, age, family history, smoking, and certain anatomical features (such as a thick neck or a large tongue). Men are also more likely than women to suffer from sleep apnea, although the risk for women increases after menopause.

Treatment
Treatment options for sleep apnea may include lifestyle changes (such as weight loss and quitting smoking), continuous positive airway pressure (CPAP) therapy, oral appliances to keep the airway open, and, in some cases, surgery. CPAP therapy

involves wearing a mask connected to a machine that delivers a steady stream of air to keep the airway open during sleep.

### 3. Restless Legs Syndrome (RLS)

Definition and Symptoms
Restless Legs Syndrome (RLS) is a neurological disorder characterized by an uncontrollable urge to move the legs, typically accompanied by uncomfortable sensations. Symptoms often worsen in the evening or at night, making it challenging to fall asleep or stay asleep. Individuals with RLS may describe sensations such as creeping, crawling, or tingling in the legs.

Causes
The exact cause of RLS is often unknown, but it can be linked to genetics, iron deficiency, chronic diseases (such as diabetes and kidney failure), and certain medications. Pregnant women may also experience RLS, particularly during the third trimester.

Treatment
Management of RLS often includes lifestyle changes, such as regular exercise, maintaining a regular sleep schedule, and avoiding caffeine and alcohol. Iron supplements may be recommended if iron deficiency is a factor. In more severe cases, medications may be prescribed to help alleviate symptoms.

## 4. Narcolepsy

Definition and Symptoms
Narcolepsy is a chronic sleep disorder characterized by excessive daytime sleepiness and sudden sleep attacks that occur at inappropriate times. Individuals with narcolepsy may experience cataplexy—sudden loss of muscle tone triggered by strong emotions, such as laughter or surprise. Other symptoms include sleep paralysis and hallucinations during the transition between wakefulness and sleep.

Causes
The exact cause of narcolepsy is not fully understood, but it is believed to involve genetic factors and abnormalities in the brain's regulation of sleep-wake cycles. A deficiency in hypocretin, a neurotransmitter that helps regulate wakefulness, has also been linked to narcolepsy.

Treatment
While there is no cure for narcolepsy, treatments can help manage symptoms. Stimulant medications are often prescribed to help improve wakefulness during the day, while antidepressants may help control cataplexy. Behavioral strategies, such as scheduled naps and maintaining a regular sleep schedule, can also be beneficial.

## 5. Circadian Rhythm Disorders

Definition and Symptoms

Circadian rhythm disorders occur when the body's internal clock is misaligned with the external environment, leading to sleep difficulties. Common types include delayed sleep phase disorder (DSPD), where individuals struggle to fall asleep and wake up at socially acceptable times, and shift work disorder, which affects individuals who work non-traditional hours.

Causes

These disorders can be caused by lifestyle factors, such as irregular sleep schedules or exposure to light at night, and can significantly impact daily functioning. Shift work, travel across time zones, and irregular sleep patterns can disrupt the natural circadian rhythm.

Treatment

Management strategies for circadian rhythm disorders may include light therapy, melatonin supplementation, and maintaining consistent sleep schedules. For those with DSPD, gradually shifting sleep times and exposure to bright light in the morning can help reset the internal clock.

## Conclusion 3

Sleep disorders are prevalent and can significantly impact an individual's health and quality of life. Recognizing the signs and symptoms of these disorders is the first step toward seeking effective treatment. By understanding the underlying causes and available interventions, individuals can take proactive measures to improve their sleep and overall well-being. In the following chapters, we will delve deeper into specific strategies for enhancing sleep hygiene, managing stress, and addressing the psychological factors that contribute to sleep disturbances.

# Chapter 4: Sleep Hygiene Practices

Sleep hygiene refers to the practices and habits that promote consistent, uninterrupted sleep. Developing good sleep hygiene is essential for optimizing sleep quality and improving overall well-being. This chapter outlines effective sleep hygiene practices, the underlying principles behind them, and how they can help mitigate sleep disturbances.

## 1. Maintain a Consistent Sleep Schedule

Importance of Routine

One of the most critical components of sleep hygiene is establishing a consistent sleep schedule. Going to bed and waking up at the same time every day helps regulate your body's internal clock (circadian rhythm), making it easier to fall asleep and wake up naturally.

Tips for Implementation

- Set a Sleep Schedule: Choose a bedtime and wake-up time that allows for 7-9 hours of sleep and stick to it, even on weekends.

- Create a Pre-Sleep Routine: Engage in relaxing activities before bedtime, such as reading, taking a warm bath, or practicing mindfulness. This signals to your body that it's time to wind down.

## 2. Optimize Your Sleep Environment

Creating a Sleep-Friendly Space

The environment in which you sleep plays a significant role in sleep quality. A conducive sleep environment is dark, quiet, and cool.

Tips for an Optimal Sleep Environment

- Control Light: Use blackout curtains or an eye mask to block out light. Minimize exposure to screens (phones, computers, TVs) at least an hour before bed, as blue light can interfere with melatonin production.

- Minimize Noise: Consider using earplugs, white noise machines, or soothing sounds to drown out disruptive noises.

- Maintain a Comfortable Temperature: The ideal bedroom temperature is generally between 60-67°F (15-19°C). Adjust bedding and sleepwear to ensure comfort throughout the night.

## 3. Be Mindful of Food and Drink

Impact of Diet on Sleep
What you consume, particularly in the hours leading up to bedtime, can significantly affect sleep quality. Certain foods and beverages can disrupt sleep, while others may promote relaxation.

Tips for Healthy Eating Habits

- Limit Caffeine and Nicotine: Avoid consuming caffeine (found in coffee, tea, chocolate, and some sodas) and nicotine (found in tobacco products) in the late afternoon and evening, as they are stimulants that can disrupt sleep.

- Avoid Heavy Meals: Large or rich meals close to bedtime can cause discomfort and indigestion. Aim to have dinner at least two to three hours before going to bed.

- Consider Sleep-Promoting Snacks: If you're hungry before bed, opt for sleep-promoting snacks like bananas, oatmeal, or yogurt, which contain nutrients that support sleep.

## 4. Engage in Regular Physical Activity

Benefits of Exercise
Regular physical activity is associated with improved sleep quality and duration. Exercise helps reduce stress, anxiety, and depression, all of which can interfere with sleep.

Guidelines for Exercise

- Aim for Consistency: Strive for at least 150 minutes of moderate-intensity aerobic activity each week, such as walking, cycling, or swimming.

- Timing Matters: While exercise is beneficial for sleep, try to avoid vigorous workouts close to bedtime. Aim to finish exercising at least three hours before sleep to prevent disruptions.

## 5. Manage Stress and Anxiety

The Link Between Stress and Sleep
High levels of stress and anxiety can lead to racing thoughts and an inability to relax, making it challenging to fall asleep. Managing stress is vital for promoting restful sleep.

Stress-Reduction Techniques

- Practice Mindfulness and Relaxation: Incorporate relaxation techniques into your pre-sleep routine, such as deep breathing, meditation, or progressive muscle relaxation.

- Keep a Journal: Writing down your thoughts and concerns before bed can help clear your mind and alleviate anxiety.

- Seek Professional Support: If stress and anxiety are overwhelming, consider speaking with a mental health professional for additional support and coping strategies.

### 6. Limit Naps

The Impact of Napping
While short naps can be beneficial, excessive daytime napping can interfere with nighttime sleep, particularly if taken too late in the day.

Guidelines for Napping

- Keep Naps Short: Limit naps to 20-30 minutes to reduce the risk of sleep inertia (grogginess upon waking) and nighttime sleep disruption.

- Timing is Key: If you need to nap, aim to do so earlier in the afternoon to minimize its impact on nighttime sleep.

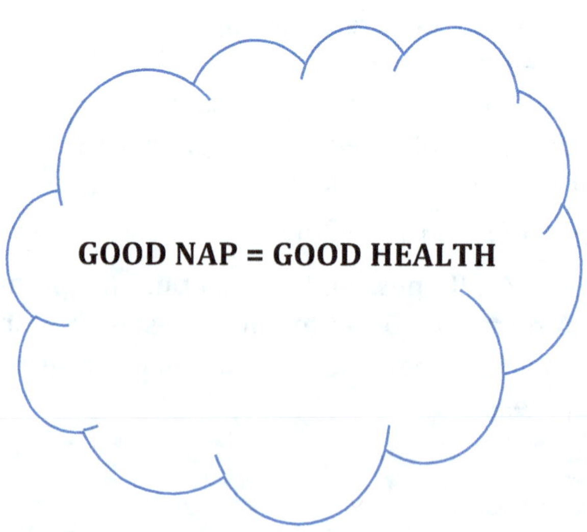

## 7. Be Mindful of Substance Use

Effects of Substances on Sleep
Certain substances, including alcohol and recreational drugs, can disrupt sleep architecture and lead to fragmented sleep patterns.

Guidelines for Responsible Use

- Limit Alcohol Intake: While alcohol may initially help you fall asleep, it often disrupts sleep later in the night and can worsen sleep quality.

- Avoid Recreational Drugs: Be cautious with the use of recreational drugs, as many can have long-term effects on sleep quality and overall health.

**Conclusion 4**

Incorporating good sleep hygiene practices into your daily routine can significantly enhance your sleep quality and overall health. By establishing consistent sleep patterns, creating a conducive sleep environment, being mindful of your diet, engaging in physical activity, managing stress, and limiting substance use, you can take proactive steps toward achieving restful and restorative sleep. In the following chapters, we will explore the psychological aspects of sleep, including the impact of mental health on sleep quality and effective strategies for overcoming sleep-related challenges.

| LIFE STAGE | DAILY SLEEP NEEDS |
| --- | --- |
| **NEWBORNS** (0–3 MONTHS) | 14–17 hours |
| **INFANTS** (4–11 MONTHS) | 12–15 hours |
| **TODDLERS** (1–2 YEARS) | 11–14 hours |
| **PRESCHOOLERS** (3–5 YEARS) | 10–13 hours |
| **SCHOOL AGE** (6–13 YEARS) | 9–11 hours |
| **TEENAGERS** (14–17 YEARS) | 8–10 hours |
| **YOUNGER ADULTS** (18–25) | 7-9 hours |
| **ADULTS** (26–64) | 7-9 hours |
| **OLDER ADULTS** (65+) | 7-8 hours |

# Chapter 5: The Psychological Aspects of Sleep

Sleep is not merely a biological necessity; it is also deeply intertwined with our psychological well-being. Our mental state can significantly influence sleep quality, and conversely, sleep disturbances can exacerbate psychological issues. This chapter explores the intricate relationship between sleep and mental health, including how psychological factors can impact sleep patterns and vice versa.

## 1. The Connection Between Sleep and Mental Health

Understanding the Bidirectional Relationship Research has established a bidirectional relationship between sleep and mental health. Poor sleep can contribute to the development of mental health disorders, such as anxiety, depression, and bipolar disorder. Conversely, pre-existing mental health issues can lead to sleep disturbances, creating a vicious cycle that affects overall health and quality of life.

- Insomnia and Depression: Studies show that individuals with chronic insomnia are at a higher risk of developing depression. The lack of restorative sleep can exacerbate feelings of sadness and hopelessness.

- Anxiety Disorders and Sleep: Anxiety often leads to racing thoughts and restlessness, making it challenging to fall asleep. Conversely, insufficient sleep can heighten anxiety levels, leading to increased worry and stress.

## 2. Stress and Its Impact on Sleep

The Role of Stress
Stress is one of the most significant contributors to sleep disturbances. When the body perceives stress, it activates the fight-or-flight response, releasing stress hormones such as cortisol. Elevated cortisol levels can disrupt sleep cycles, leading to difficulty falling asleep, staying asleep, or waking too early.

Stress Management Techniques

- Mindfulness and Meditation: Practicing mindfulness and meditation can help reduce stress levels and promote relaxation, making it easier to fall asleep.

- Cognitive Behavioral Therapy (CBT): CBT techniques can help individuals identify and change negative thought patterns associated with stress, leading to improved sleep quality.

## 3. The Role of Emotions in Sleep Quality

Emotional Regulation and Sleep
Emotions play a crucial role in sleep quality. Unregulated emotions, such as anger, sadness, or fear, can interfere with the ability to relax and fall asleep. Individuals may find themselves ruminating on negative emotions, leading to heightened arousal and difficulty winding down at night.

Strategies for Emotional Regulation

- Journaling: Writing about emotions and experiences can help process feelings and reduce anxiety before bedtime.

- Expressive Therapies: Engaging in art, music, or dance therapy can help individuals express and process emotions, promoting relaxation and better sleep.

### 4. The Impact of Cognitive Patterns on Sleep

Negative Thought Patterns
Cognitive distortions, such as catastrophizing or overgeneralizing, can create excessive worry and anxiety, leading to sleep disturbances. For example, an individual may worry excessively about not getting enough sleep, which ironically makes it more difficult to fall asleep.

Cognitive Behavioral Strategies

- Cognitive Restructuring: This technique involves identifying and challenging negative thought patterns, replacing them with more positive or realistic thoughts. For example, instead of worrying about the consequences of not sleeping, one might focus on the strategies they can implement to improve sleep.

- Sleep Restriction Therapy: This CBT technique limits the amount of time spent in bed to increase sleep efficiency. By restricting time in bed, individuals may feel more tired and find it easier to fall asleep.

### 5. The Influence of Lifestyle Factors on Sleep

Lifestyle and Sleep Patterns
Several lifestyle factors, including diet, exercise, and screen time, can impact sleep quality. Poor lifestyle choices can contribute to stress and anxiety, further affecting sleep.

Promoting Healthy Lifestyle Changes

- Balanced Diet: Consuming a diet rich in nutrients can support overall mental health and improve sleep quality. Foods high in tryptophan, magnesium, and omega-3 fatty acids can promote relaxation and better sleep.

- Physical Activity: Regular physical activity has been shown to improve mood and reduce anxiety, leading to better sleep quality. However, it's essential to time exercise appropriately to avoid interfering with sleep.

## 6. The Role of Sleep Disorders in Mental Health

Co-occurrence of Sleep Disorders and Mental Health Issues
Many individuals with sleep disorders also experience mental health issues. For example, those with insomnia are at a higher risk of developing anxiety and depression. Similarly, conditions like sleep apnea can lead to cognitive impairments, mood changes, and increased risk of depression.

Integrated Treatment Approaches

- Collaborative Care: Treating sleep disorders in conjunction with mental health issues can lead to better outcomes. For example, individuals with insomnia may benefit from both CBT-I and antidepressant medications.

- Holistic Approaches: Incorporating mindfulness, stress management, and lifestyle changes into treatment plans can help address both sleep

disturbances and mental health issues
simultaneously.

## Conclusion 5

The psychological aspects of sleep are complex and multifaceted. Understanding the interplay between sleep and mental health can empower individuals to take proactive steps toward improving both their sleep quality and overall well-being. By recognizing the impact of stress, emotions, and cognitive patterns on sleep, individuals can develop effective strategies to enhance their sleep hygiene and address underlying psychological issues. In the following chapters, we will delve into specific techniques for overcoming sleep challenges and enhancing overall sleep quality.

---

# Chapter 6: Overcoming Sleep Challenges

Despite the importance of good sleep hygiene and an understanding of the psychological aspects of sleep, many individuals still face challenges that disrupt their ability to achieve restorative sleep. This chapter explores common sleep challenges, their causes, and effective strategies to overcome them.

## 1. Insomnia

Understanding Insomnia
Insomnia is one of the most prevalent sleep disorders, characterized by difficulty falling asleep, staying asleep, or waking up too early. It can be acute (short-term) or chronic (long-term), significantly affecting overall health and well-being.

Causes of Insomnia

- Stress and Anxiety: Daily stressors, major life changes, and anxiety can all contribute to insomnia.

- Medical Conditions: Chronic pain, respiratory issues, and other medical conditions can interfere with sleep.

- Poor Sleep Habits: Inconsistent sleep schedules, excessive screen time, and stimulants can all contribute to insomnia.

Strategies for Overcoming Insomnia

- Cognitive Behavioral Therapy for Insomnia (CBT-I): This structured program helps individuals identify and change thoughts and behaviors that contribute to sleep problems. Techniques include stimulus control, sleep restriction, and cognitive restructuring.

- Sleep Environment Optimization: Create a calming sleep environment that promotes relaxation. Ensure your bedroom is dark, cool, and quiet, and invest in comfortable bedding.

- Relaxation Techniques: Engage in relaxation exercises, such as deep breathing, progressive muscle relaxation, or guided imagery, before bedtime to calm the mind.

## 2. Sleep Apnea

Understanding Sleep Apnea
Sleep apnea is a serious sleep disorder characterized by repeated interruptions in breathing during sleep. It often leads to fragmented sleep and can result in daytime fatigue, mood disturbances, and cognitive impairments.

Causes of Sleep Apnea

- Obstructive Sleep Apnea (OSA): This occurs when the muscles at the back of the throat relax excessively during sleep, blocking the airway.

- Central Sleep Apnea (CSA): This type occurs when the brain fails to send proper signals to the muscles that control breathing.

- Risk Factors: Factors such as obesity, age, and anatomical features (e.g., enlarged tonsils) can increase the risk of sleep apnea.

Strategies for Overcoming Sleep Apnea

- Weight Management: For individuals with OSA, losing weight can significantly reduce the severity of the condition and improve sleep quality.

- Continuous Positive Airway Pressure (CPAP) Therapy: This common treatment involves wearing a mask connected to a machine that delivers a continuous flow of air, keeping the airway open during sleep.

- Lifestyle Changes: Avoid alcohol and sedatives, as these can relax throat muscles and worsen sleep apnea. Sleeping on one's side rather than the back can also help.

### 3. Nightmares and Night Terrors

Understanding Nightmares and Night Terrors Nightmares are distressing dreams that often result in awakening and difficulty returning to sleep. Night terrors, more common in children, involve sudden awakening with intense fear, screaming, and confusion, often without memory of the event.

Causes of Nightmares and Night Terrors

- Stress and Anxiety: High levels of stress, trauma, or anxiety can trigger nightmares.

- Sleep Deprivation: Lack of sleep can lead to more frequent and intense nightmares.

- Certain Medications: Some medications, particularly antidepressants and sleep aids, may increase the likelihood of experiencing nightmares.

Strategies for Overcoming Nightmares and Night Terrors

- Establish a Relaxing Pre-Sleep Routine: Incorporate calming activities before bed to reduce stress and anxiety, such as reading, meditation, or gentle yoga.

- Address Underlying Stressors: If nightmares are linked to stress or trauma, consider seeking therapy or counseling to address these underlying issues.

- Imagery Rehearsal Therapy: This technique involves visualizing a positive outcome for recurring nightmares during waking hours, which can help reduce their frequency.

## EEG RECORDINGS DURING SLEEP

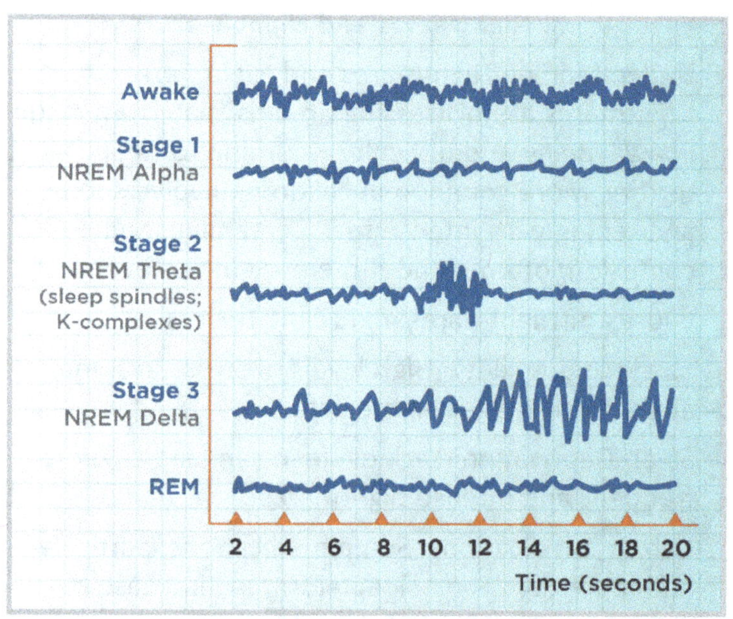


**Pic credit: Lumen Learning**

## 4. Circadian Rhythm Disorders

Understanding Circadian Rhythm Disorders
Circadian rhythm disorders occur when the body's internal clock is out of sync with the external environment. This can lead to difficulties falling asleep and waking at appropriate times.

Types of Circadian Rhythm Disorders

- Delayed Sleep Phase Disorder (DSPD): Individuals with DSPD struggle to fall asleep until late at night and have difficulty waking up in the morning.

- Advanced Sleep Phase Disorder (ASPD): Individuals with ASPD feel the urge to sleep early in the evening and wake up very early.

- Shift Work Disorder: This occurs in individuals who work non-traditional hours, leading to misalignment between their work schedule and the natural sleep-wake cycle.

Strategies for Overcoming Circadian Rhythm Disorders

- Light Exposure: Increasing exposure to natural light during the day can help regulate the circadian rhythm. Conversely, reducing light exposure in the evening can signal the body that it's time to wind down.

- Melatonin Supplementation: For some individuals, melatonin supplements can help regulate sleep-wake cycles, especially for those with delayed sleep phase disorder.

- Consistent Sleep Schedule: Establish a regular sleep schedule, even on weekends, to help reset the internal clock.

## 5. Sleep-Related Movement Disorders

Understanding Sleep-Related Movement Disorders
These disorders involve involuntary movements during sleep, which can disrupt sleep quality.

Common types include Restless Legs Syndrome (RLS) and Periodic Limb Movement Disorder (PLMD).


Causes of Sleep-Related Movement Disorders

- RLS: Often linked to genetics, iron deficiency, and certain chronic conditions.

- PLMD: Involves repetitive movements, such as kicking or twitching, during sleep without the associated sensations of RLS.


Strategies for Overcoming Sleep-Related Movement Disorders

- Lifestyle Modifications: Engaging in regular physical activity, avoiding caffeine and nicotine, and managing stress can help reduce symptoms.

- Medical Treatment: In some cases, medications may be prescribed to alleviate symptoms, particularly for those with severe RLS or PLMD.

## Conclusion 6

Overcoming sleep challenges requires a multifaceted approach that considers individual circumstances and underlying causes. By understanding the nature of specific sleep disorders and implementing effective strategies, individuals can improve their sleep quality and overall health. The next chapters will focus on the importance of sleep in physical health and cognitive function, further highlighting why prioritizing sleep is essential for a balanced and healthy life.

# *Sleep: The Hidden Strength by OTHER AUTHORS

*Sleep* is crucial for maintaining physical, mental, and emotional well-being. Scientists from various fields have studied its importance, offering diverse perspectives:

---

1. Sleep as a Cognitive Enhancer

Dr. Matthew Walker, a renowned neuroscientist and author of *Why We Sleep*, emphasizes that:

- Sleep consolidates memories by transferring short-term memories in the hippocampus to long-term storage in the cortex.

2. Sleep and Physical Health

Dr. Allan Rechtschaffen, a pioneer in sleep research, discovered that:

- Sleep deprivation weakens the immune system and makes the body more susceptible to illness.

3. Emotional Regulation Through Sleep

Dr. Rosalind Cartwright, also known as the "Queen of Dreams," studied the impact of sleep on emotional health.

- Sleep allows the brain to process and regulate emotions by connecting them with past experiences during REM sleep.

This page is a reference for other books on sleep psychology. CONTINUE >

# Chapter 7: The Importance of Sleep for Physical Health

Sleep plays a crucial role in maintaining physical health. It is during sleep that the body engages in restorative processes essential for growth, repair, and overall well-being. This chapter explores the various ways in which sleep impacts physical health, including its effects on the immune system, cardiovascular health, metabolic function, and more.

## 1. Sleep and the Immune System

The Role of Sleep in Immune Function
Adequate sleep is vital for a healthy immune system. During sleep, the body produces cytokines, proteins that help regulate immune responses. Sleep deprivation can lead to reduced production of these proteins, making individuals more susceptible to infections.

Research Findings

- Increased Illness Risk: Studies show that individuals who do not get enough sleep are more likely to catch colds and suffer from infections. A study conducted by the University of California, San Francisco, found that participants who slept less than seven hours per night were three times more likely to develop a cold than those who slept eight hours or more.

- Vaccine Efficacy: Sleep quality has also been linked to the effectiveness of vaccinations. Research indicates that individuals who are well-rested produce a stronger immune response to vaccines compared to those who are sleep-deprived.

## 2. Sleep and Cardiovascular Health

Understanding the Connection
Sleep is closely linked to cardiovascular health. Insufficient sleep can lead to increased blood pressure, inflammation, and other risk factors associated with heart disease.

Research Findings

- Hypertension: Chronic sleep deprivation is associated with higher levels of hypertension, or high blood pressure. A meta-analysis published in the journal *Sleep* found that individuals who reported short sleep duration had a significantly higher risk of developing hypertension.

- Heart Disease: Research has shown that inadequate sleep can lead to an increased risk of heart disease, heart attacks, and strokes. The American Heart Association identifies poor sleep as a risk factor for cardiovascular disease.

## 3. Sleep and Metabolic Function

The Impact of Sleep on Metabolism

Sleep is essential for maintaining metabolic health. Disruptions in sleep can affect hormones that regulate appetite and metabolism, leading to weight gain and an increased risk of obesity and type 2 diabetes.

Research Findings

- Hormonal Imbalance: Lack of sleep affects levels of ghrelin (the hunger hormone) and leptin (the satiety hormone). Sleep-deprived individuals tend to have higher levels of ghrelin and lower levels of leptin, which can lead to increased appetite and cravings for unhealthy foods.

- Insulin Resistance: Studies indicate that insufficient sleep can lead to insulin resistance, a precursor to type 2 diabetes. A study published in the journal *Diabetes Care* found that participants who experienced sleep deprivation had a significantly higher risk of developing insulin resistance.

### 4. Sleep and Weight Management

The Relationship Between Sleep and Weight Quality sleep is crucial for weight management. Sleep deprivation can alter metabolic processes and lead to unhealthy eating habits, ultimately resulting in weight gain.

Research Findings

- Increased Caloric Intake: Research shows that sleep-deprived individuals tend to consume more calories, particularly from high-carbohydrate and high-fat foods. A study published in the *American Journal of Clinical Nutrition* found that participants who were sleep-deprived consumed an average of 300 more calories per day than those who were well-rested.

- Exercise Performance: Inadequate sleep can impair physical performance and recovery, making it challenging to engage in regular exercise—a critical factor in weight management. Studies have shown that athletes who do not get enough sleep may experience decreased endurance, strength, and reaction time.

## 5. Sleep and Hormonal Balance

Understanding Hormonal Regulation
Sleep plays a crucial role in regulating various hormones, including stress hormones, growth hormones, and sex hormones. Disruptions in sleep can lead to hormonal imbalances that negatively impact overall health.

Research Findings

- Cortisol Levels: Chronic sleep deprivation is associated with elevated levels of cortisol, the stress hormone. High cortisol levels can lead to increased anxiety, weight gain, and other health issues.

- Growth Hormone Release: Sleep is the primary time for the release of growth hormone, which plays a vital role in tissue growth and muscle repair. Inadequate sleep can impair recovery from exercise and hinder muscle growth.

# 6. Sleep and Aging

The Role of Sleep in Healthy Aging
As individuals age, sleep patterns often change, and many older adults experience sleep disturbances. However, maintaining good sleep hygiene is essential for healthy aging.

Research Findings

- Cognitive Function: Sleep plays a critical role in maintaining cognitive function as individuals age. Studies have shown that poor sleep quality is associated with an increased risk of cognitive decline and dementia.

- Physical Health: Adequate sleep is essential for maintaining physical health in older adults. It supports immune function, helps manage chronic conditions, and contributes to overall quality of life.

**Conclusion 7**

Sleep is a cornerstone of physical health, impacting everything from the immune system to metabolic function. Understanding the importance of sleep can motivate individuals to prioritize their sleep hygiene and make necessary lifestyle changes. By recognizing the intricate relationship between sleep and physical health, individuals can take proactive steps to improve their sleep quality and, in turn, enhance their overall well-being. The next chapter will delve into the importance of sleep for cognitive function, highlighting how sleep influences memory, learning, and overall brain health.

---

## Chapter 8: The Importance of Sleep for Cognitive Function

Cognitive function encompasses various mental processes, including memory, attention, problem-solving, and decision-making. Sleep plays a vital role in supporting these cognitive functions, and its impact on the brain cannot be overstated. This chapter explores how sleep affects cognitive performance, learning, memory consolidation, and overall brain health.

## 1. Sleep and Memory

The Role of Sleep in Memory Formation
Sleep is essential for both the formation of new memories and the consolidation of existing ones. Memory formation occurs in three stages: encoding, storage, and retrieval, and sleep is critical during the storage phase.

Research Findings

- Memory Consolidation: During sleep, particularly during rapid eye movement (REM) sleep, the brain processes and organizes information acquired throughout the day. A study published in the journal *Nature* found that participants who took a nap after learning new information performed better on recall tests than those who remained awake.

- Declarative and Procedural Memory: Sleep enhances different types of memory. Declarative memory (facts and information) benefits from slow-wave sleep (SWS), while procedural memory (skills and tasks) improves with REM sleep. Research indicates that individuals who have adequate sleep after learning new skills perform significantly better compared to those who are sleep-deprived.

## 2. Sleep and Attention

The Impact of Sleep on Attention and Focus Adequate sleep is crucial for maintaining attention and focus. Sleep deprivation can lead to significant impairments in cognitive processes, including attention span, reaction time, and decision-making abilities.

Research Findings

- Reduced Attention Span: Studies have shown that sleep-deprived individuals exhibit decreased attention and vigilance. A study published in the journal *Sleep* found that participants who had restricted sleep performed poorly on attention tasks compared to those who had adequate sleep.

- Increased Errors: Lack of sleep can result in increased errors in tasks requiring attention and concentration. For instance, research indicates that sleep-deprived individuals are more likely to make mistakes in simple tasks, impacting performance in academic and occupational settings.

### 3. Sleep and Problem-Solving

Understanding Problem-Solving Skills
Sleep plays a critical role in enhancing problem-solving skills and creativity. The brain's ability to make connections and generate new ideas is significantly influenced by sleep quality.

Research Findings

- Enhanced Creativity: Studies have shown that individuals who are well-rested are more likely to think creatively and develop innovative solutions to problems. REM sleep, in particular, has been linked to enhanced creative thinking and problem-solving abilities.

- Insight and Aha Moments: Sleep has been associated with the phenomenon known as "insight" or "Aha moments." Research indicates that taking breaks or sleeping on a problem can led to sudden realizations or solutions that might not be evident when fully awake. A study published in *Psychological Science* found that participants who napped after engaging in problem-solving tasks demonstrated greater insight compared to those who remained awake.

### 4. Sleep and Emotional Regulation

The Relationship Between Sleep and Emotions
Sleep has a significant impact on emotional regulation and mental health. Insufficient sleep can lead to heightened emotional reactivity, increased anxiety, and mood disorders.

Research Findings

- Emotional Reactivity: Sleep deprivation can lead to greater emotional responses and reduced ability to regulate emotions. Studies show that individuals who are sleep-deprived are more likely to react negatively to stressors and exhibit mood swings.

- Risk of Mental Health Disorders: Chronic sleep deprivation has been linked to an increased risk of mental health disorders, including anxiety and depression. Research indicates that individuals with insomnia or poor sleep quality are more likely to experience symptoms of anxiety and depression.

### 5. Sleep and Cognitive Decline

Understanding the Link Between Sleep and Cognitive Decline

Quality sleep is essential for maintaining cognitive function as individuals age. Poor sleep patterns are associated with an increased risk of cognitive decline and neurodegenerative diseases.

Research Findings

- Alzheimer's Disease: Studies have found a correlation between sleep disturbances and an increased risk of Alzheimer's disease. Sleep plays a role in the brain's ability to clear amyloid plaques, which are associated with the development of Alzheimer's. Research published in *Nature Communications* indicated that individuals with disrupted sleep patterns had higher levels of amyloid buildup in the brain.

- Cognitive Impairment: Longitudinal studies have shown that individuals with poor sleep quality are at a higher risk of developing cognitive impairment and dementia as they age. A study published in the journal *JAMA Neurology* found that individuals with chronic sleep issues were more likely to experience cognitive decline over time.

## 6. Sleep and Learning

The Impact of Sleep on Learning Efficiency
Sleep is essential for effective learning and retention of information. Adequate sleep enhances the ability to absorb and process new information, leading to improved learning outcomes.

Research Findings

- Learning New Information: Research shows that sleep helps with the assimilation of new information learned during the day. A study published in the journal *Cognitive Neuroscience* found that participants who had a full night's sleep after learning performed significantly better in recalling new information compared to those who were sleep-deprived.

- Active Learning: Sleep also facilitates active learning. Engaging in sleep-dependent learning techniques, such as spaced repetition and review before sleep, can enhance memory retention and recall.

## Conclusion 8

Sleep is not merely a passive state of rest but a critical component of cognitive function. Its impact on memory, attention, problem-solving, emotional regulation, and learning underscores the importance of prioritizing quality sleep for mental performance and overall well-being. The next chapter will focus on Creating Healthy Sleep Habits, providing practical strategies to enhance sleep quality and promote better health.

Sleep is the silent architect of our strength, rebuilding what the day has worn down and preparing us to rise anew.

-Rohan Sahoo

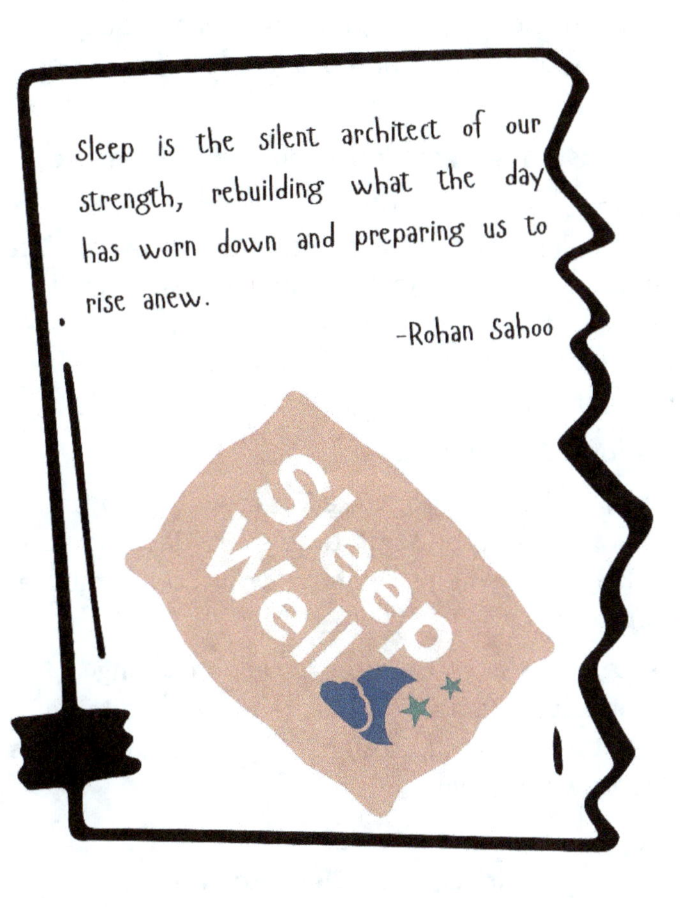

## Chapter 9: Creating Healthy Sleep Habits

Creating healthy sleep habits is essential for maximizing the benefits of sleep on physical health, cognitive function, and emotional well-being. This chapter outlines strategies for establishing a consistent sleep routine, improving sleep quality, and overcoming common barriers to restful sleep.

### 1. Establishing a Consistent Sleep Schedule

The Importance of Routine
Maintaining a regular sleep schedule helps regulate the body's internal clock, making it easier to fall asleep and wake up at the desired times. A consistent sleep routine can significantly improve sleep quality.

Tips for Consistency

- Set a Fixed Sleep and Wake Time: Aim to go to bed and wake up at the same time every day, even on weekends. This helps reinforce your body's natural sleep-wake cycle.

- Create a Pre-Sleep Routine: Develop calming activities before bed, such as reading, meditating, or gentle stretching, to signal to your body that it's time to wind down.

### 2. Optimizing the Sleep Environment

Creating a Sleep-Friendly Space
The environment in which you sleep can greatly impact sleep quality. Optimizing your sleep environment involves making adjustments to lighting, temperature, noise levels, and bedding.

Tips for an Ideal Sleep Environment

- Control Light Exposure: Keep your bedroom dark by using blackout curtains or eye masks. Avoid screens from phones, tablets, or computers at least an hour before bed, as blue light can disrupt melatonin production.

- Maintain a Comfortable Temperature: The ideal bedroom temperature for sleep is typically between 60-67°F (15-19°C). Adjust your thermostat or use fans or blankets to achieve comfort.

- Minimize Noise: Use white noise machines or earplugs to block out disruptive sounds. Consider adding soft background music or nature sounds if they help you relax.

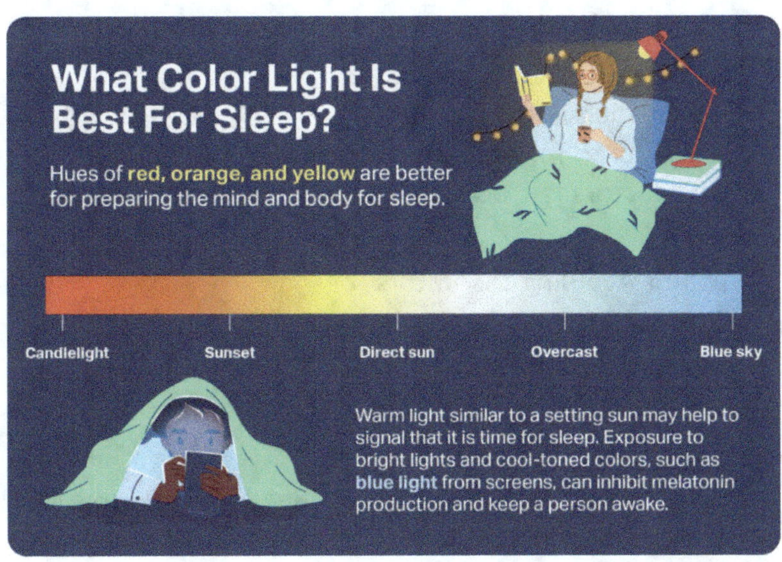


**pic credit: Sleep Foundation**

### 3. Practicing Relaxation Techniques

Managing Stress and Anxiety
Incorporating relaxation techniques into your nightly routine can help ease stress and anxiety, making it easier to fall asleep.

Tips for Relaxation

- Mindfulness and Meditation: Engage in mindfulness practices or meditation before bed. Even just a few minutes of focused breathing can help calm the mind.

- Progressive Muscle Relaxation: This technique involves tensing and then relaxing each muscle group in the body, promoting physical relaxation and signaling to the brain that it's time to sleep.

### 4. Limiting Stimulants and Disruptors

Avoiding Sleep Disruptors
Certain substances and behaviors can interfere with the ability to fall and stay asleep. Being mindful of these factors is crucial for maintaining healthy sleep habits.

Tips for Avoiding Disruptors

- Limit Caffeine and Nicotine: Reduce or eliminate caffeine and nicotine intake in the hours leading up to bedtime, as these stimulants can interfere with sleep quality.

- Avoid Heavy Meals and Alcohol: Refrain from large meals or alcohol consumption close to bedtime. While alcohol may initially make you feel drowsy, it can disrupt sleep later in the night.

## 5. Incorporating Movement and Exercise

The Benefits of Physical Activity
Regular physical activity can promote better sleep by helping to reduce stress and anxiety, as well as tiring the body in a healthy way.

Tips for Exercise

- Find the Right Time: Aim to engage in regular exercise, ideally earlier in the day. Exercising too close to bedtime may have the opposite effect and make it harder to fall asleep.

- Choose Activities You Enjoy: Whether it's walking, running, yoga, or dancing, choose activities that you enjoy to make it easier to stay consistent.

## 6. Utilizing the 8×3 Law for Sleep Optimization

Understanding the 8×3 Law
The 8×3 Law by Rohan Sahoo emphasizes the importance of managing time effectively throughout the day. This concept can be applied to enhance sleep habits as well. The idea is to allocate time wisely, focusing on eight essential tasks within three-hour intervals. Here's how you can apply it to your sleep routine:

- Prioritize Sleep as One of Your Essential Tasks: Treat sleep as a critical task that requires dedicated time. Ensure you allocate sufficient time for restful sleep within your 8×3 framework.

- Implement Breaks and Relaxation Periods: Incorporate short breaks throughout your day to reduce stress and mental fatigue. Use these intervals for mindfulness practices or light physical activity, which can promote better sleep at night.

- Create Evening Downtime: As you approach the end of your day, allow yourself a three-hour window for winding down. This can include leisure activities, preparing for the next day, and engaging in relaxing routines to signal to your body that it's time to sleep.

*Rohan Sahoo's 8×3 Law is a groundbreaking guide to mastering time management in a way that aligns with modern challenges and aspirations. Drawing inspiration from behavioral science and productivity principles, Rohan introduces a practical framework to optimize daily routines while maintaining balance and focus.

---

The Concept: What Is the 8×3 Law?

The 8×3 Law is built on the idea of dividing the 24 hours of a day into three focused blocks of 8 hours each:

1. 8 Hours of Important Tasks: Dedicated to meaningful work, study, or pursuits that align with long-term goals.

2. 8 Hours of Unimportant/Soft Tasks: Allocated for less critical activities, relaxation, or tasks that do not demand intense focus.

3. 8 Hours of Rest: Reserved for sleep and mental recovery to recharge for the next day.

The law emphasizes structure and intentionality in time use, ensuring that every hour contributes to personal growth, well-being, or productivity.

## Conclusion 9

By implementing these strategies and techniques, individuals can cultivate healthy sleep habits that enhance their overall well-being. Remember that sleep is a vital component of physical health, cognitive function, and emotional balance. Prioritizing quality sleep not only improves daily performance but also contributes to long-term health benefits. Embracing the 8×3 Law can further help in organizing your time effectively, ensuring that sleep remains a top priority in your daily routine.

As Rohan Sahoo wisely puts it, *"Managing your time effectively is just as crucial as managing your sleep. Both are essential for achieving a balanced and fulfilling life."* By respecting your sleep needs and integrating them into your daily schedule, you can unlock your full potential.

---

## Final Conclusion

As we conclude this exploration into the world of sleep and its profound impact on our lives, it's essential to remember that quality sleep is not merely a luxury but a fundamental component of overall health. The insights gathered in this book serve as a guide to understanding sleep's significance, identifying the flaws in our sleep habits, and implementing strategies to overcome them. By prioritizing sleep, we can unlock our full potential, improve our cognitive function, and enhance our emotional well-being.

## About the Author

**Rohan Sahoo**, a passionate advocate for personal growth and well-being, is dedicated to helping individuals recognize the importance of effective time management and the vital role sleep plays in achieving a balanced life. As a graduate in commerce and an author, Rohan's work reflects his commitment to exploring the intersections of psychology, health, and personal development. His unique approach combines practical strategies with insightful theories, encouraging readers to take control of their lives through better sleep and mindful time management.

## Acknowledgments

I would like to express my heartfelt gratitude to everyone who has supported me throughout the journey of writing this book. Thank you to my family and friends for their unwavering encouragement and understanding during the writing process. A special thanks to my mentors and colleagues who have inspired me with their insights on psychology and well-being.

I would also like to acknowledge the researchers and psychologists whose work has informed this book. Their contributions to the field of sleep science have been invaluable, and I hope this book helps spread their important findings to a wider audience.

# A Note to the Reader

*Dear Reader,*

*Thank you for taking the time to read this book. I hope you have found the information helpful and inspiring. Sleep is a journey, and each step you take towards improving your sleep habits is a step towards a healthier and more fulfilling life. Remember, it's never too late to make positive changes.*

*As you embark on this journey, I encourage you to be patient with yourself. Creating new habits takes time, and setbacks are a natural part of the process. Embrace the journey of self-discovery, and allow the insights from this book to guide you toward better sleep and improved well-being.*

*Wishing you restful nights and brighter days ahead.*

*Warm regards,*
*Rohan Sahoo*

# A Broad Chart on Sleep Cycle (explained from Chapter 1)

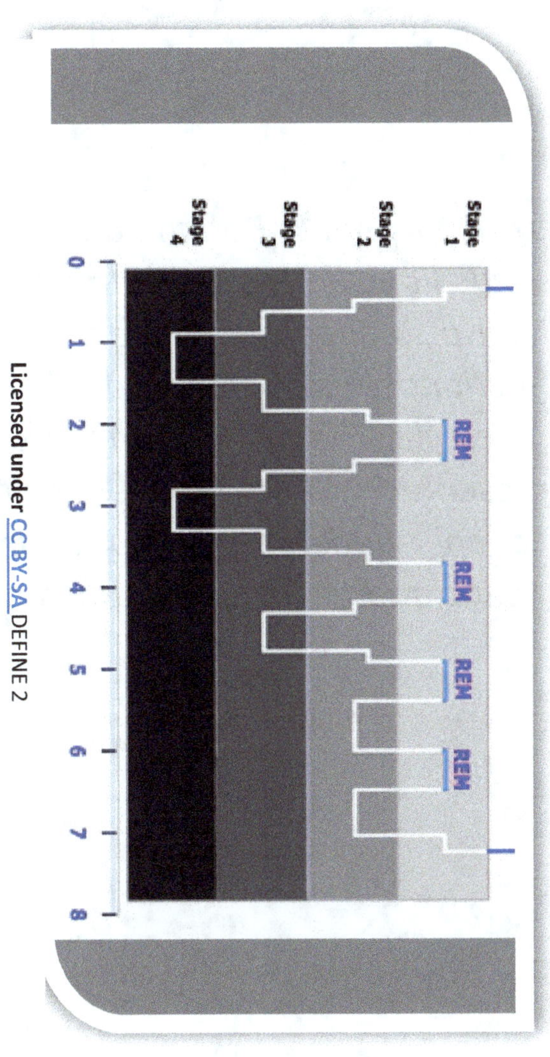

# FINAL THOUGHTS

*With this book, Rohan Sahoo not only sheds light on the importance of sleep but also encourages readers to take actionable steps toward a healthier lifestyle. The insights and strategies presented will help readers cultivate a deeper understanding of their sleep needs and embrace the power of rest in their daily lives.*

**P.S.** *It's just the beginning of the great.*

# ABOUT AUTHOR's LIFE

**Deepmanyu Sahoo** (pen name: Rohan Sahoo) is an inspiring author, commerce graduate, and creative force dedicated to exploring personal growth, storytelling, and innovation. Deepmanyu hails from a vibrant background rooted in academic curiosity and artistic expression. With a profound passion for unraveling life's complexities, he has written thought-provoking works that span genres, from time management and business strategies to heartfelt novellas and thrilling supernatural tales.

Beyond writing, Deepmanyu is a key creator of **DJEASTRE**, where he contributes as a music director and label manager, showcasing his versatility and creative flair. His work with, alongside a talented team, demonstrates his dedication to building meaningful projects in both literature and music.

His life is a tapestry of creativity, discipline, and exploration. From crafting timeless love stories and delving into the intricacies of sleep science to contributing to his community with remote classes in Badagada Brit Colony, he embodies the spirit of innovation and empathy. His books and projects, including works like *8×3 Law* and *Recharge: The Silent Power of Sleep*, reflect his mission to inspire others to prioritize their well-being and embrace purposeful living.

At the heart his journey is his ability to blend art, science, and storytelling to create work that resonates deeply with his audience, leaving a lasting impact on their lives.

* 9 7 9 8 3 0 3 8 8 4 8 4 7 *